15 IMPRESSIVE WAYS TO LOWER CHOLESTEROL

A must practice reducing cholesterol at all times

By

Dr. DOUGLAS JASON

TABLE OF CONTENT

ABOUT THE AUTHOR

INTRODUCTION

ABOUT THE AUTHOR

Dr. Douglas Jason is a certified dietician who has a strong passion for wellness and a big eagerness to help people all over the world. He uses healthy food, herbs, spices, and other useful tools to help mankind realize its overall goal of optimum health.

INTRODUCTION

Easy Ways to Reduce Cholesterol
A change in diet and lifestyle can help lower your cholesterol range when you have a high cholesterol level. It has been demonstrated that lowering cholesterol lowers the risk of heart disease. Diet and exercise, in addition to taking a cholesterol-lowering prescription, can promote the healthiest heart and blood vessel function. The following

advice includes easy techniques to maintain good health.

CHAPTER 1

PORTION CONTROL.

The body needs a certain amount of cholesterol to function properly. However, levels of LDL "bad" cholesterol are increased by both dietary saturated fat and cholesterol. High LDL cholesterol levels can result in artery plaque buildup, which can cause heart disease and stroke. Because it aids in the removal of harmful cholesterol from circulation, HDL is a "good" cholesterol. You can change your diet to lower LDL cholesterol and increase HDL cholesterol.

Employ Your Hand
Large meal portions are linked to weight gain and high cholesterol. Using your hand as a measuring device for portions is a simple approach to practicing portion management for a meal. About the size of one serving of food is one handful.

CHAPTER 2

Serve up heart-healthy food.

Pick up the pace when it comes to fruits and vegetables! Several meals spread out throughout the day can aid in reducing LDL "bad" cholesterol. Additionally, these meals include antioxidants, which may be advantageous. Additionally, eating more fruits and vegetables can lead to consuming fewer high-fat items. Additionally, this can lower blood pressure and encourage weight loss.

CHAPTER 3

Think Fish For Heart Health.

Because many fish are high in heart-healthy omega-3 fatty acids and low in saturated fat, eating fish is particularly heart-healthy. Omega-3 fatty acids are what contribute to reducing triglyceride levels in the blood. Choose fatty fish, which has more omega-3, instead. Keep in mind that any deep-fried item loses some of its nutritional value.

CHAPTER 4

Start the day with whole grains.

As a result of the fiber and complex carbs in oatmeal and whole-grain cereal, you'll feel fuller for longer and be less likely to overeat in the afternoon. These breakfast options can aid in weight management and help lower LDL "bad" cholesterol.

CHAPTER 5

Go Nuts for Cardiovascular Health

Considering how abundant monounsaturated fat nuts are, they aid in lowering cholesterol. While keeping HDL "good" cholesterol levels constant, this type of fat lowers LDL "bad" cholesterol. Heart disease risk may be reduced as a result. However, limit yourself to a few as nuts contain a lot of calories, particularly if they have a chocolate or sugar coating.

CHAPTER 6

Unsaturated fats protect the heart.

Only roughly one-third of our daily caloric demands are for fat. The type of fat does matter, though. Canola, olive, and safflower oils include unsaturated fats that can lower LDL "bad" cholesterol levels. Trans fats and saturated fats (found in butter and palm oil) raise LDL cholesterol. Every fat contains calories. Using moderation is crucial.

CHAPTER 7

Eat fewer potatoes and more beans

Carbohydrates are crucial for the generation of energy. However, there are variations in caloric quality as well. Whole grains rich in fiber, such as beans, quinoa, whole-wheat pasta, and brown rice, can decrease cholesterol. Additionally, whole grains prolong your feeling of fullness. Pastries, white rice, white bread, and potatoes are high in carbs, which quickly raise blood sugar levels. You may become more hungry as a result, which could result in overeating.

CHAPTER 8

Get Moving with Exercise

Regular, short bursts of exercise can raise HDL cholesterol and reduce triglycerides. By assisting you in preserving a healthy body weight, exercise also enhances cardiovascular health. It can assist you in maintaining a healthy weight, which lowers your risk of high pressure and heart disease. One non-drug method of lowering cholesterol through food is this.

CHAPTER 9

Just go for a walk,

All you need is a good pair of shoes to start walking, which is simple and beneficial. Walking can also help you lose weight, keep your balance, and maintain strong bones while lowering your risk of heart disease and stroke. Don't be frightened to start there; short walks are preferable to no walks. As your body gains strength, you can progressively work your way up to longer walks.

CHAPTER 10

Work Out Without Visiting the Gym

Any cardiovascular exercise is good for your heart. But for recommendations, consult your physician. Gardening, dancing, or choosing the stairs over the elevator are a few easy activities that can be beneficial. Exercise can even include household chores.

CHAPTER 11

Take Charge of Your Health

Learn the strategies that will keep your health in check so you can stay on track with a reliable cholesterol management program. It can be quite beneficial to check the nutrition statistics on food labels. To keep you engaged and motivated, it might also be beneficial to change up your exercise routine.

CHAPTER 12

What to Do When Dining Out,

Be mindful of the caliber and size of your meal when dining out. Beware of calories, saturated fats, and hidden salt. Avoid placing oversized orders. Instead of frying your meals, opt for broiled, baked, steamed, and grilled options. So that you may decide how much sauce you want, request it on the side.

CHAPTER 13

Watch Out for Hidden Traps

The process of lowering cholesterol through diet starts at the grocery store. Examine the nutrition facts. Verify the serving sizes. Do single-serve packages have two servings rather than just one? Select foods that are low in trans fat and high in saturated fat.

CHAPTER 14

Don't worry.

Stress can significantly increase your cholesterol level. Additionally, raising blood pressure has the potential to cause heart and blood vessel illness. Reducing stress can be enjoyable. Take a vacation from your typical everyday activities. Meditation, biofeedback, and relaxation techniques are all easy and efficient ways to lower stress.

Chapter 15:

When You Lose, You Win.

When you lose weight, you reduce your risk of stroke and heart disease as well as blood pressure, cholesterol, and triglycerides. The heart is less stressed when the body is at its ideal weight. Additionally, it lessens the tension on ligaments and joints.

CONCLUSIONS

Observe Your Physician's Advice
Maintain a normal cholesterol range
for the rest of your life by visiting the
doctor frequently, exercising, and
eating a balanced diet. You can
increase longevity and lower your
risk of disease by making these
lifestyle modifications. Consult your
medical providers for advice on how
to modify your routine to lower your
cholesterol